Breast Health

Breast health is crucial for women, and it involves understanding breast self-examination, screening for breast cancer, and maintaining overall breast wellness. Awareness of breast health and early detection of abnormalities are key in improving outcomes and reducing mortality rates.

MCQUEEN MATT

Copyright

McQueen Matt

Breast Health

© 2023, McQueen Matt

Self-published

Mhizta.matt@gmail.com

Table of Content

Introduction 2

Chapter One..7

    Breast Self-Examination (BSE).................................7

Chapter Two 12

    Clinical Breast Examination (CBE) 12

Chapter Three 16

    Mammography 16

Chapter Four..19

    Breast Cancer Awareness 19

Chapter 5 23

    Healthy lifestyle choices 23

Conclusion 27

Table of Figures

Fig.1 Breast Self-Examination 10

Fig.2 Clinical Breast Examination 16

Fig.3 Mammography..20

Fig.4 Mammography Result..21

Fig.5 Breast Cancer Awareness..24

Breast Health

Introduction

Breast health refers to the overall well-being and care of the breasts, which are an important part of a woman's body. It involves maintaining the normal structure and function of the breasts while being aware of any changes or abnormalities that may indicate potential health issues. Regular breast self-examination is a crucial component of breast health, allowing women to become familiar with the normal look and feel of their breasts and promptly detect any changes such as lumps, skin changes, or nipple discharge. By being proactive in self-monitoring, women can play an active role in maintaining their breast health.

In addition to breast self-examination, clinical breast examinations by healthcare professionals are recommended as part of routine check-ups. These examinations involve a thorough assessment of the breasts to detect any signs of abnormalities. Regular mammograms, which are X-ray screenings for breast cancer, are also important for early detection. Mammograms can often detect breast cancer before it can be felt or noticed, leading to earlier intervention and improved outcomes. Women should follow the recommended screening guidelines based on their age and individual risk factors.

Promoting breast health also extends to adopting a healthy lifestyle. Regular exercise, a balanced diet rich in fruits and vegetables, limited alcohol consumption, and avoidance of smoking contribute to overall well-being, including breast health. These healthy lifestyle choices can help reduce the risk of developing breast cancer and other breast-related conditions.

Overall, maintaining breast health involves a combination of self-awareness, regular screenings, and healthy lifestyle practices. By staying vigilant, being proactive in self-examination, and seeking appropriate medical care, women can prioritize their breast health and improve their chances of early detection and effective management of any potential breast-related concerns.

Breast health encompasses various aspects that contribute to the well-being and care of a woman's breasts. It involves understanding the normal anatomy and function of the breasts and being aware of any changes or abnormalities that may indicate potential health issues. Regular breast self-examination is an essential practice for maintaining breast health. By becoming familiar with the normal look and feel of their breasts, women can quickly identify any changes such as new lumps, changes in size or shape, skin dimpling, nipple discharge, or other unusual symptoms. Prompt detection of such changes allows for timely medical evaluation and intervention, potentially catching any issues at an early stage.

Clinical breast examinations performed by healthcare professionals are also vital for maintaining breast health. During these examinations, a healthcare provider carefully examines the breasts for any signs of abnormalities, including palpable lumps or unusual tissue changes. These examinations, typically conducted as part of routine check-ups or in response to specific concerns, complement self-examination by providing a trained eye and expertise in evaluating breast health.

In addition to self-examination and clinical assessments, mammography plays a crucial role in breast health. Mammograms are specialized X-ray screenings that can detect breast cancer at an early stage, often before any noticeable symptoms arise. These regular screenings are recommended based on age and individual risk factors and are essential for early detection and treatment of breast cancer, potentially saving lives and improving outcomes.

It is important to note that maintaining breast health extends beyond regular screenings and examinations. Adopting a healthy lifestyle can contribute to overall breast health and reduce the risk of breast-related issues. Engaging in regular physical activity, maintaining a balanced diet, limiting alcohol consumption, and avoiding smoking are all important factors in promoting breast health and reducing the risk of breast cancer.

In summary, breast health involves being knowledgeable about the normal appearance and feel of the breasts, conducting regular self-examinations, undergoing clinical breast examinations, and following recommended mammogram screening guidelines. Additionally, adopting a healthy lifestyle further supports breast health. By prioritizing breast health through awareness, self-care practices, and medical screenings, women can take proactive steps towards maintaining their well-being and early detection of any potential breast-related concerns.

Chapter One
Breast Self-Examination (BSE)

Breast self-examination is a simple technique that women can perform on themselves to become familiar with the normal look and feel of their breasts. By regularly examining their breasts, women can detect any changes or abnormalities such as lumps, changes in size or shape, skin dimpling, or nipple discharge. BSE should ideally be done monthly, a few days after the end of menstruation.

Breast Self-Examination (BSE) is a practice that allows women to actively monitor their breast health by checking for any changes or abnormalities. It involves a systematic examination of the breasts using one's own hands and eyes. BSE is typically performed once a month and serves as an important complement to regular clinical breast examinations and mammograms.

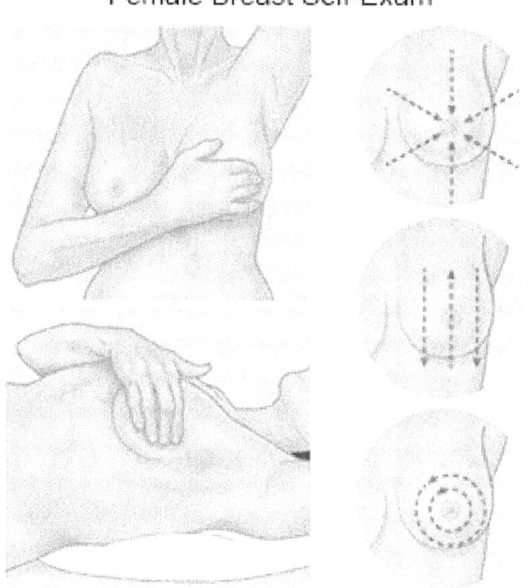

Fig.1 Breast Self-Examination

During BSE, a woman visually inspects her breasts for any changes in size, shape, or skin texture. By observing in front of a mirror and raising the arms, she can identify any visible abnormalities or asymmetry between the breasts. The next step involves lying down and using the pads of the fingers to systematically feel the breast tissue. Using circular motions, gentle pressure is applied to check for any lumps, thickening, or other unusual findings.

The purpose of BSE is to promote breast awareness and early detection of potential issues. By becoming familiar with the normal look and feel of the breasts, women can promptly detect any changes that may require further medical evaluation. It is important to note that BSE is not a diagnostic tool and cannot replace clinical examinations or mammograms. However, it empowers women to actively participate in their breast health and seek timely medical attention if any abnormalities are detected. Regular BSE, in combination with other screening methods, contributes to overall breast health and aids in early detection of breast-related concerns.

Here is an explanation of how to perform BSE:

1. Choose a convenient time: BSE should ideally be performed once a month, a few days after the end of menstruation when the breasts are less likely to be tender or swollen.

When it comes to performing Breast Self-Examination (BSE), choosing a convenient time refers to selecting the right moment in your menstrual cycle for optimal comfort and ease. It is generally recommended to perform BSE a few days after the end of menstruation. During this time, the breasts are less likely to be tender, swollen, or sensitive, which can make the examination more comfortable and easier to perform.

By choosing a convenient time in your menstrual cycle, you can minimize discomfort and enhance the accuracy of your self-examination. It is important to note that if you have reached menopause or have an irregular menstrual cycle, you can choose any time of the month to perform BSE.

By being mindful of the timing, you can ensure that you can perform the examination with greater ease and potentially detect any changes or abnormalities in your breasts more effectively. Remember, the goal is to establish a regular routine for self-examination and maintain breast health throughout the year.

2. Observe in front of a mirror: Stand in front of a mirror with your arms relaxed at your sides. Inspect your breasts visually for any changes in size, shape, or skin texture. Look for any visible lumps, dimpling, redness, or nipple abnormalities.

3. Raise your arms: Raise your arms overhead and observe your breasts' appearance in different positions. Pay attention to any changes or asymmetry between the two breasts.

4. Lie down and examine with your fingers: Lie down flat on your back and place a pillow or towel under your right shoulder. Use the pads of your three middle fingers on your left hand to gently explore your right breast in a circular motion, starting from the outer edge and moving towards the nipple. Cover the entire breast, including the upper and lower areas, and use light, medium, and firm pressure while feeling for any lumps or abnormalities.

5. Repeat for the other breast: After examining the right breast, move the pillow or towel to your left shoulder and repeat the same circular motion with your right hand to examine your left breast.

6. Check the nipples: Gently squeeze each nipple and check for any discharge or changes in shape or color.

If you notice any changes, such as new lumps, thickening, swelling, dimpling, changes in nipple appearance, or any other unusual symptoms, it is important to consult with a healthcare professional for further evaluation. Remember, BSE is not a substitute for clinical breast examinations and mammograms but serves as an important tool for self-awareness and early detection of potential breast issues. Regular breast self-examinations, along with clinical assessments and mammograms as recommended, can contribute to maintaining breast health and detecting any concerns in a timely manner.

Chapter Two

Clinical Breast Examination (CBE)

Clinical Breast Examination (CBE): Clinical breast examination involves a healthcare professional examining the breasts for any signs of abnormalities. It is typically recommended as a part of routine check-ups and is important for early detection of potential issues.

Clinical Breast Examination (CBE) is a physical examination of the breasts performed by a healthcare professional, such as a doctor or nurse. It is a vital component of routine check-ups and plays a crucial role in assessing breast health, detecting abnormalities, and ensuring early detection of potential breast-related issues.

During a CBE, the healthcare provider will carefully examine the breasts and surrounding areas for any signs of abnormalities, such as lumps, changes in texture or skin color, nipple changes, or other unusual findings. The examination usually involves visual inspection and palpation (feeling) of the breasts and the areas under the arms.

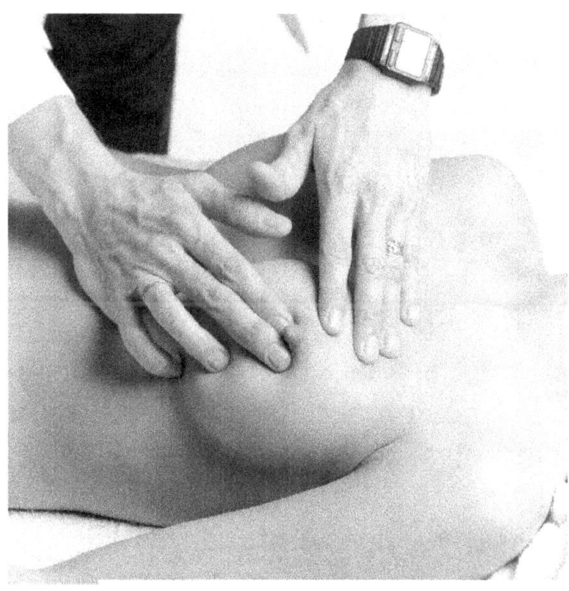

Fig.2 Clinical Breast Examination

The healthcare provider may use their fingers to systematically assess the breast tissue, checking for any lumps or irregularities. They may vary the pressure applied to feel different layers of tissue and ensure thorough examination. The examination also includes checking the lymph nodes in the underarm area, as these can be an important indicator of breast health. They will typically use different levels of pressure and cover the entire breast area, including the outer edges, inner regions, and under the armpits. This thorough examination helps identify any abnormalities that may be present deep within the breast tissue.

CBE allows for a trained professional to evaluate breast health and detect any potential abnormalities that may require further investigation, such as imaging tests like mammograms or ultrasound. It complements self-examination and provides an additional level of assessment by someone with expertise in recognizing signs of breast-related issues.

Clinical Breast Examination is an important part of regular healthcare visits for women, and it is recommended at different intervals depending on factors such as age, risk factors, and individual health history. It is an integral aspect of breast health management, alongside self-examination and mammography, contributing to early detection and improved outcomes in breast-related concerns.

Clinical Breast Examination serves as a valuable tool for assessing breast health, particularly in combination with other screening methods such as self-examination and mammography.

It allows for the expertise and experience of a healthcare professional to be applied in evaluating breast tissue and detecting any potential abnormalities that may require further investigation or follow-up.

Early detection of breast-related issues through CBE can significantly improve treatment outcomes and contribute to overall breast health. It is recommended that women undergo regular CBE as part of their comprehensive healthcare routine

Chapter Three
Mammography

Mammography is a specific type of X-ray imaging that is used to screen for breast cancer in women who have no apparent symptoms. It can detect breast cancer at an early stage, often before it can be felt or noticed. Regular mammograms are recommended based on age and individual risk factors.

Mammography is a specialized imaging technique that uses low-dose X-rays to examine the breasts for any signs of breast cancer or other abnormalities. It is an essential screening tool for the early detection of breast cancer in women, even before any noticeable symptoms appear. Mammograms can detect breast changes that may indicate cancer long before they can be felt during a clinical breast examination or by the woman herself.

During a mammogram, the woman's breast is gently compressed between two plates to spread out the breast tissue and obtain clear images. The compression may cause temporary discomfort but is necessary for proper imaging. The breast is imaged from different angles to capture multiple views and provide a comprehensive assessment of the breast tissue.

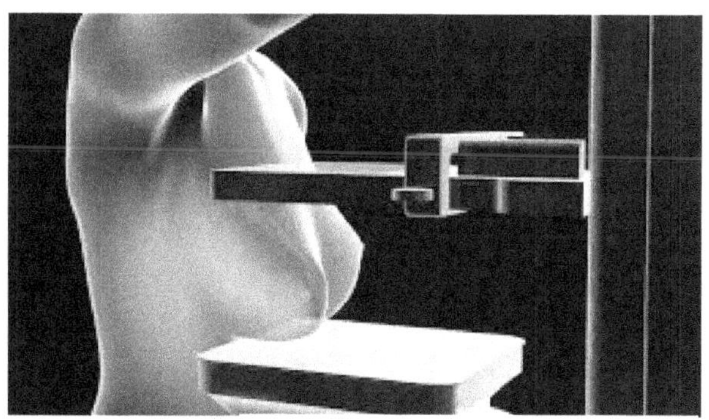

Fig.3 Mammography

The images obtained during a mammogram are examined by radiologists, who are specialized doctors trained to interpret these images. They look for any signs of abnormalities, such as masses, calcifications, or distortions in the breast tissue. If an abnormality is detected, further evaluation, such as additional imaging tests or a biopsy, may be recommended to determine whether the abnormality is benign or cancerous.

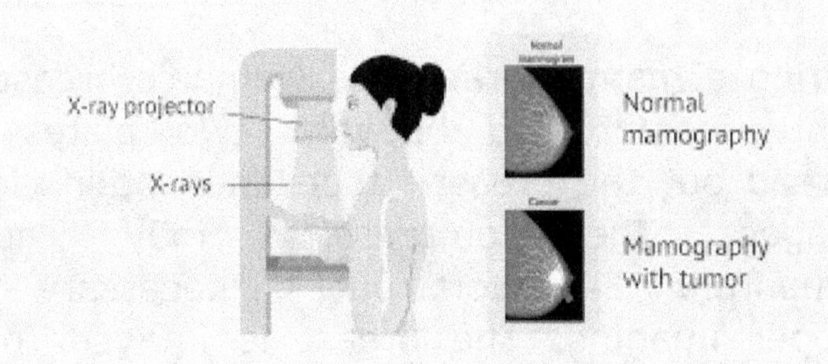

Fig.4 Mammography Result

Mammography plays a crucial role in breast cancer screening and has been proven to reduce mortality rates by detecting breast cancer at an early stage when it is more treatable. Regular mammograms are recommended based on age and individual risk factors. Generally, women between the ages of 40 and 74 are advised to undergo mammograms every one to two years. However, recommendations may vary depending on personal and family history of breast cancer, genetic factors, and other risk factors.

It's important to note that mammography is not perfect and may not detect all breast cancers. However, it remains the most widely used and effective tool for early detection and screening of breast cancer. It is crucial for women to discuss their specific screening recommendations with their healthcare providers to determine the appropriate frequency and timing of mammograms based on their individual risk profile.

Chapter Four
Breast Cancer Awareness

Breast cancer is the most common cancer among women worldwide. Raising awareness about breast cancer risk factors, signs and symptoms, and the importance of early detection is crucial. This includes educating women about the significance of mammograms, regular check-ups, and genetic testing for individuals with a family history of breast cancer.

Breast Cancer Awareness refers to efforts and initiatives aimed at increasing public knowledge and understanding about breast cancer, its risks, symptoms, and the importance of early detection and treatment. The objective of Breast Cancer Awareness campaigns is to raise awareness, educate the public, promote early screening, and support individuals affected by breast cancer.

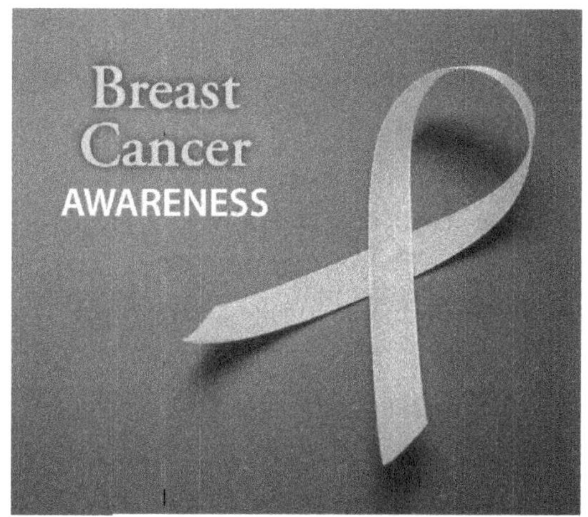

Fig.5 Breast Cancer Awareness

Breast cancer is the most common cancer among women worldwide, and awareness campaigns play a vital role in empowering individuals to take proactive steps in managing their breast health. These initiatives typically take place during Breast Cancer Awareness Month, which is observed in October globally. However, breast cancer awareness activities occur throughout the year to ensure a continuous focus on prevention, education, and support.

Breast Cancer Awareness campaigns aim to:

1. Educate about risk factors and prevention: These campaigns provide information about the risk factors associated with breast cancer, such as age, family history, genetic mutations, hormonal factors, and lifestyle choices. They emphasize the importance of adopting a healthy lifestyle, including regular exercise, maintaining a balanced diet, limiting alcohol consumption, and avoiding smoking. Educational materials, workshops, and community events help individuals understand how they can reduce their risk of developing breast cancer.

2. Promote early detection: Early detection is crucial for improving breast cancer outcomes. Breast Cancer Awareness campaigns emphasize the importance of regular self-examination, clinical breast examinations by healthcare professionals, and mammography screenings. They provide information on how to perform breast self-examinations and encourage women to be aware of any changes in their breasts and seek medical attention promptly if any abnormalities are detected.

3. Support individuals affected by breast cancer: Breast Cancer Awareness initiatives focus on providing support, resources, and information for individuals diagnosed with breast cancer and their loved ones. They promote support networks, survivor stories, counseling services, and educational materials to help patients navigate their journey, make informed decisions, and access appropriate medical care and emotional support.

Breast Cancer Awareness campaigns use various platforms and strategies to reach a wide audience. These include media campaigns, public service announcements, fundraising events, educational workshops, social media campaigns, and partnerships with healthcare organizations, advocacy groups, and community organizations. The goal is to engage individuals, dispel myths and misconceptions surrounding breast cancer, and empower people with accurate information and resources.

By raising awareness about breast cancer risks, symptoms, and the importance of early detection and treatment, Breast Cancer Awareness initiatives strive to save lives, support patients, and promote a world where breast cancer is diagnosed at early stages when treatment options and survival rates are more favorable.

Chapter 5
Healthy lifestyle choices

Maintaining a healthy lifestyle can contribute to breast health. This includes regular exercise, a balanced diet rich in fruits and vegetables, limiting alcohol consumption, and avoiding smoking. These lifestyle choices can help reduce the risk of developing breast cancer and improve overall well-being.

Healthy lifestyle choices refer to conscious decisions and behaviors that promote physical, mental, and emotional well-being. These choices encompass various aspects of life, including nutrition, physical activity, sleep, stress management, and avoiding harmful substances. Adopting a healthy lifestyle is essential for overall health and can significantly reduce the risk of chronic diseases, improve quality of life, and enhance longevity.

1. Nutrition: Making healthy food choices is crucial for maintaining a balanced diet and providing the body with essential nutrients. A healthy diet includes a variety of fruits, vegetables, whole grains, lean proteins, and healthy fats. It is important to limit the intake of processed foods, added sugars, unhealthy fats, and excessive salt.

2. Physical activity: Regular physical activity is essential for maintaining a healthy weight, improving cardiovascular health, strengthening muscles and bones, and enhancing overall fitness. Engaging in activities such as brisk walking, jogging, cycling, swimming, or strength training can help meet recommended exercise guidelines. Aim for at least 150 minutes of moderate-intensity aerobic activity or 75 minutes of vigorous-intensity aerobic activity per week, along with muscle-strengthening exercises at least twice a week.

3. Sleep: Prioritizing adequate sleep is vital for overall health and well-being. Aim for 7-9 hours of quality sleep each night. Establishing a consistent sleep routine, creating a comfortable sleep environment, and practicing good sleep hygiene habits can promote better sleep quality.

4. Stress management: Chronic stress can have detrimental effects on physical and mental health. It is important to find healthy ways to manage and cope with stress, such as practicing relaxation techniques (e.g., deep breathing, meditation, yoga), engaging in hobbies, seeking social support, and maintaining a work-life balance.

5. Avoiding harmful substances: Limiting or avoiding substances that can be harmful to health is crucial. This includes avoiding tobacco products and minimizing alcohol consumption. Smoking is a major risk factor for various diseases, including cancer, cardiovascular conditions, and respiratory disorders. Alcohol consumption should be moderate, with women limiting to no more than one drink per day.

6. Regular health check-ups: Regular medical check-ups and screenings are essential for early detection and prevention of diseases. Follow recommended guidelines for screenings such as mammograms, Pap smears, cholesterol checks, and blood pressure monitoring based on age, gender, and individual risk factors.

Making healthy lifestyle choices is a lifelong commitment that requires discipline, consistency, and self-care. It is important to remember that small, sustainable changes can have a significant impact on overall health and well-being. By adopting healthy habits, individuals can enjoy a higher quality of life, reduce the risk of chronic diseases, and promote a healthier future.

Conclusion

Breast health is of utmost importance for women's overall well-being. Regular monitoring, awareness, and proactive measures are essential in maintaining optimal breast health. Early detection plays a crucial role in improving outcomes for breast-related concerns, particularly breast cancer.

Breast self-examination (BSE) is a valuable tool that empowers women to become familiar with the normal look and feel of their breasts, allowing them to promptly detect any changes or abnormalities. However, it should be complemented with clinical breast examinations (CBE) conducted by healthcare professionals and mammography screenings for a comprehensive approach to breast health.

Awareness campaigns and initiatives promoting breast cancer awareness serve as a catalyst for education, early detection, and support. By disseminating accurate information, encouraging regular screenings, and offering resources for those affected by breast cancer, these campaigns contribute to saving lives and improving the quality of life for individuals facing breast-related challenges.

Healthy lifestyle choices, including proper nutrition, regular physical activity, adequate sleep, stress management, and avoiding harmful substances, are vital components of maintaining overall breast health. These choices, combined with regular check-ups and screenings, help reduce the risk of breast-related diseases and promote overall well-being.

Remember, breast health is a lifelong commitment that requires attention and care. By staying informed, being proactive, and seeking medical advice, when necessary, women can take control of their breast health and contribute to a healthier future.

www.ingramcontent.com/pod-product-compliance
Lightning Source LLC
Chambersburg PA
CBHW060905260726

48661CB00008B/3476